WALL PILATES WORKOUTS FOR WOMEN

Sculpt Your Body With Easy-To-Follow Wall Pilates Workouts For Women And Takeing On The Challenge On Embark On A 30-Day Journey With Wall Pilates Workouts For Women - Includes Training Program

CONTENTS

INTRODUCTION

Welcome to "Wall Pilates Workouts For Women," a comprehensive guide designed to revolutionize your fitness journey through the innovative practice of Wall Pilates. In this book, we delve into the transformative power of Pilates when combined with the support and resistance provided by a wall, offering a dynamic and effective approach tailored specifically for women.

A. Explanation of Wall Pilates:

Wall Pilates merges the principles of traditional Pilates with the stability and versatility of utilizing a wall as a prop. By incorporating the wall into various exercises, practitioners can enhance their alignment, stability, and strength while experiencing a unique depth in their Pilates practice. This method emphasizes controlled movements, breath awareness, and mindful engagement, fostering a deeper mind-body connection and promoting overall well-being.

B. Benefits of Wall Pilates for Women:

For women, Wall Pilates offers a multitude of benefits that cater to the unique needs and goals of the female body. From improving posture and core strength to toning muscles and enhancing flexibility, this practice provides a holistic approach to fitness. Additionally, Wall Pilates can aid in alleviating common issues such as lower back pain, pelvic floor dysfunction, and postural imbalances, making it particularly beneficial for women at all stages of life, including pregnancy and postpartum recovery.

C. Overview of the book's structure:

In "Wall Pilates Workouts For Women," we present a structured and progressive series of workouts designed to meet women's fitness goals and needs. The book is divided into sections that cater to different aspects of fitness, including core strength, flexibility, balance, and overall body conditioning. Each section features detailed instructions, accompanied by illustrations or photographs, to guide you through the exercises effectively. Furthermore, we provide modifications and variations to accommodate different fitness levels, ensuring that everyone can experience the transformative benefits of Wall Pilates.

Whether you're new to Pilates or seeking to deepen your practice, "Wall Pilates Workouts For Women" offers a comprehensive resource to help you achieve your fitness aspirations while cultivating strength, grace, and vitality. Get ready to embrace a new dimension of wellness and empowerment as you embark on this journey with us. Let's build strength, find balance, and unleash the power within through

the transformative practice of Wall
Pilates.

UNDERSTANDING WALL PILATES

In the world of fitness, innovation often stems from a blend of tradition and creativity. Wall Pilates is a prime example of this fusion, offering women a dynamic approach to strengthening their bodies while honoring the principles of Pilates. To truly grasp the essence of Wall Pilates, it's essential to delve into its history, evolution, and fundamental principles.

A. History and Origins of Pilates:

To understand Wall Pilates, one must first appreciate the roots of the broader Pilates method.

Developed by Joseph Pilates in the early 20th century, Pilates was initially known as Contrology, a system aimed at improving physical and mental well-being through controlled movements. Joseph Pilates believed that physical and mental health are interconnected and that a strong core—what he referred to as the "powerhouse"—is essential for overall fitness.

Originally practiced on mats, Pilates exercises focused on building strength, flexibility, and endurance without adding bulk. With its emphasis on alignment, breathing, and mindful movement, Pilates gained popularity among dancers, athletes, and individuals seeking a holistic approach to fitness.

B. Evolution of Pilates to include Wall Workouts:

As fitness trends evolve, so too does the Pilates method. The integration of walls into Pilates workouts represents a natural progression, offering practitioners new challenges and opportunities for exploration. While traditional Pilates exercises often utilize mats and specialized equipment like the reformer, Cadillac, and Wunda chair, incorporating walls into the practice adds an additional dimension to the workout.

The concept of Wall Pilates builds upon Joseph Pilates' original principles by leveraging the support and resistance provided by vertical surfaces. By utilizing the wall as a prop, practitioners can refine their alignment, deepen their stretches, and engage muscles in novel ways. From standing poses to inversions, Wall Pilates offers a diverse repertoire of movements that target the entire body while promoting stability, strength, and mobility.

C. Principles of Pilates and how they apply to Wall Workouts:

At the heart of Pilates lie a set of principles that guide its practice and distinguish it from other forms of exercise. These principles—centering, concentration, control, precision, breath, and flow—form the foundation of Wall Pilates as well.

Centering: Wall Pilates encourages practitioners to find their center of gravity and engage their core muscles, promoting stability and balance.

Concentration: By focusing on precise movements and alignment, practitioners cultivate a deeper mind-body connection, enhancing body awareness and proprioception.

Control: Wall Pilates emphasizes controlled, deliberate movements, ensuring proper form and minimizing the risk of injury.

Precision: Attention to detail is paramount in Wall Pilates, with practitioners striving for precision in each movement to maximize effectiveness and efficiency.

Breath: Proper breathing techniques are integral to Wall Pilates, facilitating relaxation, oxygenation, and the flow of movement.

Flow: Wall Pilates movements are designed to flow seamlessly from one to the next, promoting fluidity and grace in motion.

Incorporating these principles into Wall Pilates workouts not only enhances physical fitness but also fosters mindfulness, stress relief, and overall well-being.

Understanding the history, evolution, and principles of Pilates provides a solid foundation for exploring Wall Pilates as a dynamic and effective workout option for women seeking to enhance their strength, flexibility, and vitality. By embracing the fusion of tradition and innovation inherent in Wall Pilates, practitioners can embark on a journey of self-discovery and transformation, both on and off the mat.

GETTING STARTED

Congratulations on taking the first step towards incorporating Wall Pilates into your fitness routine! Before diving into the workouts, it's essential to set yourself up for success. In this chapter, we'll cover the essential equipment you'll need, how to set up your space effectively, and the safety precautions to keep in mind.

A. Essential Equipment:

1. Wall Anchor or Barre: The cornerstone of Wall Pilates workouts is the wall anchor or barre. This sturdy structure will provide support and stability during exercises like leg presses,

squats, and stretches. Ensure it's securely attached to the wall and positioned at a height that suits your comfort level.

2. Resistance Bands: These versatile tools add intensity to your workouts by providing resistance. Opt for bands of varying strengths to accommodate different exercises and skill levels. They're perfect for targeting specific muscle groups and enhancing overall strength and flexibility.

3. Yoga Mat: While not always necessary, a yoga mat can provide additional comfort and traction during floor exercises. Choose a mat with adequate thickness to

cushion your joints and prevent slipping.

4. Stability Ball: Incorporating a stability ball adds an element of challenge to your workouts, engaging your core muscles for balance and stability. It's great for exercises like ball squats, crunches, and back extensions.

5. Comfortable Clothing and Footwear: Wear breathable, stretchy clothing that allows for a full range of motion. For footwear, opt for supportive yet flexible shoes or go barefoot if you prefer.

B. Setting Up Your Space:

1. Clearing the Area: Choose a spacious, clutter-free area with enough room to move freely and safely. Remove any obstacles or hazards that may interfere with your workout.

2. Proximity to the Wall: Position yourself close enough to the wall anchor or barre to maintain proper form and alignment during exercises. Adjust the distance based on your height and reach.

3. Good Lighting: Ensure adequate lighting in your workout space to enhance visibility and prevent accidents. Natural light or well-placed lamps can create a bright and inviting atmosphere.

4. Ventilation: Proper airflow is essential for a comfortable and productive workout. Open windows or use fans to maintain a cool and ventilated environment, especially during intense sessions.

C. Safety Precautions:

1. Warm-Up: Always start your Wall Pilates session with a thorough warm-up to prepare your muscles and joints for exercise. Incorporate dynamic stretches and gentle movements to increase blood flow and flexibility.

2. Proper Form: Focus on maintaining proper form and alignment throughout each exercise to prevent injuries and

maximize effectiveness. Pay attention to cues from your instructor or follow along with instructional videos to ensure correct technique.

3. Gradual Progression: Listen to your body and progress at a pace that feels comfortable and sustainable. Avoid pushing yourself too hard or advancing too quickly, as this can lead to overexertion and potential injury.

4. Stay Hydrated: Drink plenty of water before, during, and after your workouts to stay hydrated and replenish lost fluids. Dehydration can negatively impact your performance and recovery, so make hydration a priority.

BEGINNER WALL PILATES EXERCISES

In this chapter, we'll delve into a series of beginner wall Pilates exercises designed to ease you into this invigorating practice. Whether you're a newcomer to Pilates or seeking to refresh your routine, these exercises will help you build strength, flexibility, and balance while utilizing the support of a wall.

A. Warm-Up Exercises:

Before diving into the core of your workout, it's essential to prepare your body with gentle warm-up exercises. These movements will help increase blood flow, loosen muscles, and activate key muscle groups.

1. Wall Roll-Downs:

Stand with your back against the wall, feet hip-width apart.

Slowly roll down, articulating through each vertebra, until your hands touch the floor or as far as comfortable.

Hold for a moment, then roll back up to standing, one vertebra at a time.

2. Wall Squats:

Stand facing the wall, about a foot away, with your feet hip-width apart.

Lean against the wall and slide down into a squat position, keeping your knees aligned with your ankles.

Hold for a few seconds, then push through your heels to return to standing.

B. Core Strengthening Workouts:

A strong core is fundamental to Pilates practice, providing stability and support for the entire body. These exercises will target your abdominal muscles and help you develop a solid foundation.

1. Wall Plank:

Begin in a standing position facing the wall, arms extended shoulder-width apart and palms flat against the wall.

Walk your feet back until your body forms a straight line from head to heels, engaging your core.

Hold this position for 30 seconds to one minute, focusing on maintaining proper alignment and breathing deeply.

2. Wall Crunches:

Lie on your back with your feet against the wall, knees bent at a 90-degree angle.

Place your hands behind your head, elbows wide, and engage your core.

Exhale as you lift your shoulder blades off the mat, bringing your chest towards your knees.

Inhale as you lower back down with control, keeping your lower back pressed into the mat.

C. Upper Body and Arm Exercises:

These exercises will target the muscles of your arms, shoulders, and upper back, helping to improve posture and upper body strength.

1. Wall Push-Ups:

Stand facing the wall, arms extended shoulder-width apart and palms flat against the wall at shoulder height.

Keeping your body straight, bend your elbows to lower your chest towards the wall.

Push through your palms to straighten your arms and return to the starting position.

2. Wall Angels:

Stand with your back against the wall, feet hip-width apart, and arms at your sides.

Slowly raise your arms overhead, keeping them in contact with the wall, until they form a "Y" shape.

Lower your arms back down to your sides with control, maintaining contact with the wall throughout the movement.

D. Lower Body and Leg Exercises:

Strengthening the muscles of your lower body is essential for stability, mobility, and balance. These exercises will target your glutes, thighs, and calves.

1. Wall Sit:

Lean against the wall with your back flat and feet hip-width apart.

Slide down until your thighs are parallel to the floor, knees bent at a 90-degree angle.

Hold this position for 30 seconds to one minute, focusing on engaging your quadriceps and keeping your core activated.

2. Wall Leg Lifts:

Lie on your side with your hips and shoulders against the wall, bottom arm extended for support.

Lift your top leg towards the ceiling, keeping it straight and engaging your outer thigh and glute.

Lower your leg back down with control, avoiding any swinging or momentum.

E. Cool-Down Stretches:

As you near the end of your workout, take time to stretch and lengthen your muscles, promoting relaxation and flexibility.

1. Wall Hamstring Stretch:

Lie on your back with your hips close to the wall and legs extended vertically against the wall.

Flex your feet and gently press your heels towards the ceiling, feeling a stretch in the back of your legs.

Hold for 30 seconds to one minute, breathing deeply and relaxing into the stretch.

2. Wall Chest Opener:

Stand facing away from the wall with your feet hip-width apart.

Place your palms flat against the wall at shoulder height, fingers pointing behind you.

Lean forward slightly, opening through your chest and shoulders, while keeping your spine long.

Practice these beginner wall Pilates exercises regularly to build strength, flexibility, and confidence in your practice. As you become more familiar with the movements, feel free to explore variations and progressions to challenge yourself further. Remember to listen to your body, breathe deeply, and enjoy the journey of self-discovery through Pilates.

ELEVATING YOUR PRACTICE: INTERMEDIATE AND ADVANCED WALL PILATES WORKOUTS

As you embark on your journey to elevate your Pilates practice, it's essential to build upon the foundations laid in the beginner exercises. In this chapter, we'll delve into intermediate and advanced Wall Pilates workouts, designed to challenge your strength, flexibility, balance, and stability while integrating your entire body into dynamic movements.

A. Progressions from Beginner Exercises:

Incorporating progressions from beginner exercises allows you to deepen your understanding of each movement while intensifying the challenge. Start by refining your alignment and engagement in familiar poses such as the Wall Roll Down and Wall Squat. As you become more comfortable, progress to variations that demand greater control and coordination, such as the Wall Plank with Leg Lifts or the Wall Teaser.

B. Adding Resistance and Intensity:

To take your workouts to the next level, introduce resistance and intensity into your routine. Utilize resistance bands or small hand weights to add extra challenge to exercises like the Wall Press and Wall Bridge. Experiment with tempo variations, incorporating slow, controlled movements to target specific muscle groups and ignite deep stabilizers. By gradually increasing the resistance and intensity, you'll continue to build strength and endurance while pushing your limits.

C. Incorporating Balance and Stability Challenges:

Balance and stability are integral components of a well-rounded Pilates practice. The wall provides a stable support system, allowing you to focus on honing your balance and stability without fear of falling. Challenge yourself with exercises like the Wall Single Leg Circle or the Wall Side Plank, incorporating subtle shifts in weight and position to engage stabilizing muscles and improve proprioception. As you master these challenges, explore dynamic movements that require rapid transitions and quick reflexes to further enhance your balance and stability.

D. Full Body Integration Workouts:

As you progress through intermediate and advanced exercises, focus on integrating your entire body into seamless, flowing movements. Emphasize fluid transitions between exercises, maintaining a strong connection between breath and movement. Explore full-body sequences such as the Wall Roll Up to Standing or the Wall Pike, which engage multiple muscle groups simultaneously while promoting core stability and spinal alignment. By embracing the concept of full-body integration, you'll cultivate a sense of unity and strength that extends beyond individual muscles or movements.

DESIGNING YOUR PERSONALIZED WALL PILATES TRAINING PROGRAM

In the journey towards fitness, customization is key. Just as every woman is unique, so too should be her workout routine. In this chapter, we delve into crafting a personalized Wall Pilates training program tailored to your individual needs. From setting up a weekly training schedule to incorporating progressions, let's embark on this transformative journey together.

A. Tailoring Workouts to Individual Needs:

No two bodies are exactly alike, and neither should be their workouts. Before diving into any exercise regimen, it's crucial to assess your individual needs, goals, and limitations. Are you aiming for weight loss, muscle toning, or improved flexibility? Do you have any existing injuries or health concerns that need to be taken into account?

With Wall Pilates, the versatility of exercises allows for customization to suit varying fitness levels and objectives. Whether you're a beginner or an experienced practitioner, modifications can be made to ensure each movement is both effective and safe. Remember, the beauty of Pilates lies in its adaptability, so don't hesitate to tailor the workouts to fit your unique requirements.

B. Weekly Training Schedule:

Consistency is the cornerstone of progress. To maximize the benefits of Wall Pilates, it's essential to establish a weekly training schedule that aligns with your lifestyle and commitments. Set aside dedicated time slots for your workouts, treating them as non-negotiable appointments with yourself.

When crafting your schedule, consider the principle of balance. Aim for a blend of strength, flexibility, and restorative sessions throughout the week. For instance, alternate between Wall Pilates sessions focusing on core stability, upper body strength, lower body engagement, and full-body integration. Intersperse these workouts with active recovery days or gentle stretching routines to prevent burnout and promote overall well-being.

Remember, quality trumps quantity. It's better to commit to a realistic schedule that you can maintain consistently rather than overloading yourself with excessive workouts that lead to fatigue or injury.

C. Incorporating Progressions:

Progress is the name of the game in any fitness endeavor. As you become more proficient in Wall Pilates, it's important to continually challenge your body by incorporating progressions into your routine. Progressions can take many forms, whether it's increasing the intensity of exercises, adding resistance with props like resistance bands or hand weights, or mastering advanced variations of familiar movements.

However, progression should always be gradual and mindful. Listen to your body's signals and respect its limitations. Push yourself out of your comfort zone, but never to the point of pain or discomfort. Remember, sustainable progress is built upon a foundation of patience, persistence, and proper technique.

In conclusion, designing a personalized Wall Pilates training program involves understanding your individual needs, crafting a balanced weekly schedule, and incorporating progressive challenges to foster continual growth. By embracing this holistic approach, you'll not only transform your body but also cultivate a deeper connection between mind, body, and spirit. So, let's roll out our mats and embark on this empowering journey towards strength, flexibility, and vitality.

EXERCISES FOR DIFFERENT FITNESS LEVELS

In the realm of Wall Pilates workouts for women, the spectrum of fitness levels is as diverse as the colors of a sunset. Whether you're just starting your fitness journey or you're a seasoned enthusiast looking to push your limits, there's a place for you against that sturdy wall. In this chapter, we'll delve into tailored exercises designed specifically for beginners, intermediate practitioners, and those who dare to embrace the challenge of advanced techniques.

A. Beginner's Guide:

For those stepping into the world of Wall Pilates for the first time, welcome! Your journey begins with laying down a solid foundation, ensuring proper form and technique while gradually building strength and flexibility. Here are a few beginner-friendly exercises to get you started:

1. Wall Squats: Stand with your back against the wall and feet hip-width apart. Slowly lower yourself into a squat position, sliding down the wall until your thighs are parallel to the ground. Hold for a few seconds, then push through your heels to return to the starting position.

2. Wall Push-ups: Face the wall, standing arm's length away. Place your hands flat against the wall at shoulder height. Lower your chest towards the wall by bending your elbows, then push back to the starting position.

3. Wall Plank: Assume a plank position with your forearms resting against the wall and elbows directly below your shoulders. Engage your core and keep your body in a straight line from head to heels. Hold for 30 seconds to a minute, gradually increasing as you build strength.

B. Intermediate Level Workouts:

Once you've mastered the basics and feel confident in your abilities, it's time to kick it up a notch with intermediate-level exercises. These movements will challenge your stability, endurance, and coordination, taking your Wall Pilates practice to the next level:

1. Wall Bridge: Lie on your back with your feet flat against the wall and knees bent. Pressing through your heels, lift your hips off the ground, forming a straight line from shoulders to knees. Hold for a few seconds, then lower back down with control.

2. Wall Plank with Leg Lift: Begin in a plank position with your feet against the wall. Lift one leg off the

wall, keeping it straight and parallel to the ground. Hold for a few seconds, then lower and switch legs.

3. Wall Pike: Start in a plank position with your feet against the wall. Engage your core as you lift your hips towards the ceiling, forming an inverted V shape with your body. Hold briefly, then lower back to plank position.

C. Advanced Techniques:

For the fearless souls ready to push their limits and unlock new heights of strength and flexibility, advanced Wall Pilates techniques await. These challenging exercises demand precision, control, and unwavering determination:

1. Wall Handstand: Begin in a plank position with your feet against the wall. Walk your hands back towards the wall until your body forms an L shape. Slowly kick up, using the wall for support as you balance upside down. Hold for as long as you can with control, then lower back down.

2. Wall Lunge Jumps: Stand facing away from the wall with one foot planted firmly against it. Lower into a lunge position, then explode off the ground, switching legs in mid-air and landing back in a lunge with the opposite foot

against the wall. Repeat, alternating legs with each jump.

3. Wall Split: Sit facing the wall with one leg extended straight against it and the other bent in front of you. Slowly slide your extended leg up the wall, keeping it straight, until you feel a deep stretch in your hamstring. Hold for a few seconds, then switch legs.

ADDRESSING COMMON CONCERNS

In the pursuit of fitness, it's natural to encounter obstacles along the way. Whether it's finding the time, dealing with physical limitations, or simply lacking motivation, these challenges can often derail our journey towards our health goals. However, with the right approach and a bit of determination, we can overcome these hurdles and emerge stronger and more resilient.

A. Overcoming Challenges:

Embarking on a wall Pilates workout regimen can be exciting, but it's essential to acknowledge and address the challenges that may arise. One common challenge is time constraints. Many women lead busy lives, juggling work, family, and other commitments, leaving little time for exercise. However, by prioritizing your health and scheduling dedicated workout sessions, you can carve out the time needed to reap the benefits of wall Pilates.

Another challenge is consistency. It's easy to start a new workout routine with enthusiasm, only to lose steam after a few weeks. To overcome this, set achievable goals, track your progress, and find a support system to hold you accountable. Remember, consistency is key to seeing results and maintaining long-term success.

Financial constraints may also pose a challenge for some women. Gym memberships and personal training sessions can be costly, making it difficult to access professional guidance. However, wall Pilates offers a budget-friendly alternative that requires minimal equipment, making it accessible to women of all financial backgrounds.

B. Modifications for Physical Limitations:

Physical limitations can present significant barriers to exercise, but they don't have to prevent you from reaping the benefits of wall Pilates. Whether you're recovering from an injury, managing a chronic condition, or simply dealing with the natural effects of aging, there are modifications you can make to tailor your workout to your specific needs.

For example, if you have lower back pain, you can perform wall Pilates exercises in a seated position or use additional support, such as cushions or pillows, to alleviate pressure on your spine. If you have joint issues, you can reduce the range of motion or use resistance bands to decrease the intensity of certain movements.

It's essential to listen to your body and communicate with your healthcare provider before starting any new exercise routine, especially if you have underlying health concerns. They can provide personalized recommendations and ensure that you're exercising safely and effectively.

C. Motivational Tips:

Staying motivated is often the biggest challenge when it comes to maintaining a consistent workout routine. Fortunately, there are several strategies you can employ to keep yourself motivated and on track.

Setting specific, achievable goals can provide a sense of direction and purpose to your workouts. Whether it's improving your flexibility, increasing your strength, or simply feeling more energized, having a clear objective can keep you focused and motivated.

Find activities that you enjoy and incorporate them into your wall Pilates workouts. Whether it's listening to your favorite music, practicing mindfulness, or working out with a friend, making exercise enjoyable can help you stay motivated and committed.

Celebrate your successes, no matter how small. Whether it's

mastering a challenging exercise or simply completing a workout, take the time to acknowledge your achievements and reward yourself for your hard work.

Remember, progress takes time, and setbacks are a natural part of the journey. Be kind to yourself, stay patient, and above all, stay committed to your health and well-being. With dedication and perseverance, you can overcome any obstacle and achieve your fitness goals with wall Pilates.

NUTRITIONAL GUIDANCE FOR OPTIMAL RESULTS

A. Importance of Diet in Pilates:

In the journey towards wellness and fitness, the significance of diet cannot be overstated. When it comes to Pilates, a discipline that emphasizes strength, flexibility, and mind-body connection, what you eat plays a crucial role in enhancing your performance and achieving optimal results.

Pilates workouts demand both physical and mental stamina. Proper nutrition provides the fuel your body needs to power through sessions effectively while supporting muscle recovery and growth. By nourishing your body with the right foods, you can amplify the benefits of your Pilates practice, whether your goal is to tone muscles, improve flexibility, or enhance overall well-being.

B. Meal Planning Tips:

Creating a nutrition plan tailored to complement your Pilates routine is key to maximizing your efforts. Here are some meal planning tips to support your fitness goals:

1. Prioritize Protein: Protein is essential for muscle repair and growth. Include lean sources such as chicken, fish, tofu, beans, and

lentils in your meals to support your Pilates workouts.

2. Embrace Whole Foods: Opt for whole, unprocessed foods rich in nutrients, vitamins, and minerals. Fill your plate with plenty of fruits, vegetables, whole grains, and healthy fats to fuel your body and promote overall health.

3. Balance Macronutrients: Aim for a balanced intake of carbohydrates, protein, and healthy fats to sustain energy levels throughout your workouts and aid in recovery afterward.

4. Hydrate Adequately: Proper hydration is crucial for maintaining peak performance

during Pilates sessions. Drink plenty of water throughout the day, especially before and after exercising, to stay hydrated and support muscle function.

5. Plan Ahead: Take the time to plan your meals and snacks in advance to ensure you have nutritious options readily available. This can help you avoid reaching for unhealthy choices when hunger strikes.

C. Recipes for Energy and Recovery:

Fueling your body with nutrient-dense meals and snacks is essential for optimizing your Pilates performance and promoting recovery. Here are a few energizing and nourishing recipes to incorporate into your meal plan:

1. Green Smoothie Bowl:

Ingredients:

1 cup spinach or kale

1 frozen banana

1/2 cup frozen berries

1/2 avocado

1 tablespoon chia seeds

1/2 cup almond milk

Toppings: sliced fresh fruit, granola, nuts, seeds

Instructions:

Blend spinach or kale, banana, berries, avocado, chia seeds, and almond milk until smooth. Pour into a bowl and top with your favorite fruits, granola, nuts, and seeds for added texture and flavor.

2. Quinoa Salad with Grilled Chicken:

Ingredients:

1 cup cooked quinoa

4 ounces grilled chicken breast, sliced

1 cup mixed greens

1/2 cup cherry tomatoes, halved

1/4 cup cucumber, diced

1/4 cup red onion, thinly sliced

2 tablespoons feta cheese, crumbled

1 tablespoon olive oil

1 tablespoon balsamic vinegar

Salt and pepper to taste

Instructions:

In a large bowl, combine cooked quinoa, grilled chicken, mixed greens, cherry tomatoes, cucumber, red onion, and feta cheese. Drizzle with olive oil and balsamic vinegar, then season with salt and pepper. Toss gently to combine, then serve immediately.

3. Peanut Butter Banana Protein Bites:

Ingredients:

1 cup rolled oats

1/2 cup natural peanut butter

1/4 cup honey or maple syrup

1/4 cup protein powder (optional)

1 ripe banana, mashed

1/4 cup dark chocolate chips (optional)

Instructions:

In a large bowl, mix together rolled oats, peanut butter, honey or maple syrup, protein powder (if using), mashed banana, and dark chocolate chips until well combined. Roll the mixture into bite-sized balls, then place them on a baking sheet lined with parchment paper. Refrigerate for at least 30 minutes before serving. Store any leftovers in an airtight container in the refrigerator for up to one week.

By incorporating these nutritious recipes and meal planning tips into your routine, you can optimize your Pilates workouts and support your journey towards achieving your fitness goals. Remember, nourishing your body with wholesome foods is an integral part of a balanced and healthy lifestyle.

BEYOND THE 30 DAYS

Congratulations on completing the initial 30 days of your Wall Pilates journey! As you continue your practice, it's essential to shift your focus from just completing the workouts to sustaining your progress, exploring further Pilates techniques, and incorporating Pilates into your daily life.

A. Sustaining Progress:

Sustaining progress requires consistency and commitment. Remember, Pilates is not just a short-term fix; it's a lifestyle. Reflect on the progress you've made during the first 30 days – the increased flexibility, strength, and improved posture. To sustain these gains, it's crucial to maintain a regular practice schedule. Set realistic goals for yourself, whether it's practicing Pilates three times a week or integrating shorter sessions into your daily routine.

Additionally, listen to your body. If you feel fatigued or notice any discomfort during your workouts, take a step back and modify the exercises accordingly. It's okay to challenge yourself, but it's equally important to prioritize your well-being. Pay attention to proper form and alignment to prevent injuries and maximize the benefits of each exercise.

B. Exploring Further Pilates Techniques:

Now that you've mastered the basics, it's time to explore further Pilates techniques. Pilates is a dynamic practice with endless variations and modifications to suit individuals of all fitness levels. Consider incorporating props such as resistance bands, stability balls, or foam rollers to add variety to your workouts and target different muscle groups.

Explore different Pilates styles, such as Classical Pilates, Contemporary Pilates, or Reformer Pilates, to discover what resonates with you. Each style offers unique exercises and approaches, allowing you to continuously challenge yourself and prevent boredom.

Don't be afraid to step out of your comfort zone and try new exercises or sequences. Embrace the learning process and celebrate your progress along the way. Remember, Pilates is not about perfection; it's about progress and personal growth.

C. Incorporating Pilates into Daily Life:

Pilates is not just confined to the studio – it can be integrated into your daily life in various ways. Whether you're sitting at your desk, cooking dinner, or waiting in line, there are opportunities to incorporate Pilates principles into your everyday activities.

Practice mindful breathing throughout the day, focusing on deep diaphragmatic breaths to center yourself and reduce stress. Engage your core muscles to support your spine and improve posture while sitting, standing, or walking. Take regular breaks to stretch and move your body, relieving tension and promoting circulation.

Additionally, look for opportunities to incorporate Pilates exercises into household chores or leisure activities. For example, use the wall for support while performing leg lifts or wall squats while brushing your teeth. Get creative and make Pilates a seamless part of your daily routine.

By sustaining your progress, exploring further Pilates techniques, and incorporating Pilates into your daily life, you'll continue to reap the countless benefits of this transformative practice beyond the initial 30 days. Embrace the journey, stay committed, and enjoy the ongoing evolution of your mind and body through Pilates.

EMBARKING ON THE 30-DAY CHALLENGE

A. Overview of the 30-Day Challenge:

Congratulations on taking the first step towards transforming your body and mind through the Wall Pilates Workouts 30-Day Challenge! This chapter will provide you with a comprehensive overview of what to expect during the next month as you embark on this journey towards health, strength, and vitality.

The 30-Day Challenge is designed to introduce you to the principles of Pilates while utilizing the support of a wall for added stability and resistance. Each day, you will engage in a series of targeted exercises that will work your core, improve your flexibility, and enhance your overall posture. By committing to this challenge, you are not only investing in your physical well-being but also in your mental and emotional health.

Throughout the next 30 days, you will gradually progress through different levels of difficulty, allowing your body to adapt and grow stronger with each passing workout. Whether you're a beginner or a seasoned Pilates practitioner, this challenge is tailored to accommodate all fitness levels, ensuring that everyone can reap the benefits of this transformative practice.

B. Daily Workouts and Progress Tracking:

To help you stay on track and monitor your progress, each day of the 30-Day Challenge will feature a specific workout routine outlined in this book. These workouts are designed to be concise yet effective, allowing you to easily incorporate them into your daily routine without feeling overwhelmed.

As you complete each workout, be sure to record your progress in the provided tracking sheet. Documenting your journey will not only help you stay accountable but also allow you to reflect on your achievements and see how far you've come by the end of the challenge.

Remember, consistency is key when it comes to seeing results. Even on days when you may not feel motivated, try to push through and complete the workout to the best of your ability. Every small step forward counts towards your ultimate goal of improved strength, flexibility, and well-being.

C. Tips for Staying Motivated and Consistent:

Staying motivated throughout the 30-Day Challenge may seem daunting at times, but with the right mindset and strategies, you can overcome any obstacles that come your way. Here are some tips to help you stay on track:

1. Set Clear Goals: Define what you hope to achieve by the end of the challenge and keep these goals in mind as you progress. Whether it's fitting into a favorite pair of jeans or simply feeling more confident in your own skin, having a clear vision of your objectives will fuel your motivation.

2. Find an Accountability Partner: Share your journey with a friend, family member, or online community. Having someone to hold you accountable and provide encouragement along the way can

make all the difference in staying committed to your workouts.

3. Mix It Up: Keep your workouts exciting and engaging by incorporating variety into your routine. Try different Pilates exercises, experiment with new techniques, or add music to energize your sessions.

4. Listen to Your Body: Pay attention to how your body feels and adjust your workouts accordingly. It's important to challenge yourself, but also to recognize when you need to rest and recover to prevent injury.

5. Celebrate Your Progress: Take time to celebrate your

achievements, no matter how small they may seem. Whether it's mastering a new exercise or increasing your flexibility, acknowledging your progress will boost your confidence and motivation to continue pushing forward.

By following these tips and staying committed to the 30-Day Challenge, you will not only transform your body but also cultivate a deeper sense of self-awareness and empowerment. So, lace up your sneakers, roll out your mat, and let's embark on this journey together towards a healthier, happier you!

VISUAL GUIDANCE FOR EFFECTIVE WALL PILATES WORKOUTS

Incorporating step-by-step videos and illustrations into your Wall Pilates routine can significantly enhance your experience and results. In this chapter, we'll delve into the importance of visual guidance, how to access online video libraries, and effectively utilize illustrations for easy follow-along.

A. Importance of Visual Guidance in Wall Pilates:

Visual guidance plays a pivotal role in mastering the intricacies of Wall Pilates. While verbal cues are helpful, seeing the movements demonstrated in real-time provides a clearer understanding of proper form and alignment. Through videos, you can observe the instructor's posture, movements, and breathing techniques, allowing you to replicate them accurately.

Furthermore, visual demonstrations help prevent injuries by highlighting common mistakes and offering corrections. Whether you're a beginner or seasoned practitioner, having a visual reference ensures you perform each exercise correctly, maximizing its effectiveness.

B. Accessing the Online Video Library:

To access a comprehensive library of step-by-step videos for Wall Pilates workouts, you can utilize various online platforms and resources. Many reputable fitness websites and apps offer specialized Pilates programs with detailed instructional videos tailored for different skill levels.

Additionally, subscribing to certified Pilates instructors' channels on video-sharing platforms like YouTube can provide a wealth of valuable content. Ensure the videos are from reputable sources and align with your fitness goals and level of expertise.

Investing in a subscription-based Pilates platform can also grant you access to a diverse range of workouts, including wall-specific routines. These platforms often offer structured programs, live classes, and on-demand videos, allowing you to customize your workouts according to your preferences and schedule.

C. How to Use Illustrations for Easy Follow-Along:

In addition to videos, illustrations serve as invaluable visual aids for enhancing your Wall Pilates practice. They provide a simplified, step-by-step breakdown of each exercise, making it easier to grasp the movements and transitions.

When utilizing illustrations, follow these tips for easy follow-along:

1. Study the Posture: Pay close attention to the starting and ending positions depicted in the illustrations. Focus on aligning your body accordingly to maintain proper form throughout the exercise.

2. Sequence of Movements: Follow the sequential order of movements illustrated, ensuring a smooth transition from one exercise to the next. Visualize each step before

executing it to enhance fluidity and precision.

3. Refer to Descriptions: Accompanying text descriptions or captions often accompany illustrations, providing additional guidance on technique and breathing patterns. Take the time to read through these instructions to deepen your understanding of the exercise.

4. Practice Patience: Mastery takes time, so be patient with yourself as you familiarize yourself with each exercise. Consistent practice coupled with visual guidance will gradually improve your proficiency and confidence in Wall Pilates.

THE COMPLETE GUIDE FOR WOMEN OF ALL AGES

In the journey towards fitness, there's no one-size-fits-all approach. Every woman is unique, with different fitness levels, health conditions, and goals. In this chapter, we'll delve into the art of customizing Wall Pilates workouts to cater to women of all ages and backgrounds. We'll explore how to adapt these exercises to address various health conditions, and we'll hear inspiring testimonials from women who've experienced remarkable success through their Wall Pilates journey.

A. Customizing Workouts for Different Fitness Levels:

One of the beauties of Wall Pilates is its adaptability. Whether you're a beginner taking your first steps into fitness or an experienced enthusiast looking to elevate your practice, there's a place for you in Wall Pilates.

For beginners, starting with gentle, foundational exercises is key. These may include basic wall stretches to improve flexibility, gentle core exercises to build strength, and simple balance drills to enhance stability. As beginners progress, they can gradually incorporate more challenging movements and increase the intensity of their workouts.

Intermediate practitioners can explore a wider range of exercises, incorporating variations and modifications to target specific muscle groups and enhance overall body awareness. They may experiment with incorporating props such as resistance bands or stability balls to add resistance and variety to their workouts.

Advanced practitioners, who have mastered the fundamentals of Wall Pilates, can take their practice to new heights by exploring advanced movements and sequences. These may include dynamic wall exercises that challenge coordination and agility, as well as advanced balance drills that push the limits of strength and stability.

No matter your fitness level, the key is to listen to your body and progress at a pace that feels comfortable and sustainable for you. With dedication and consistency, every woman can reap the benefits of Wall Pilates, regardless of where they are on their fitness journey.

B. Adapting Wall Pilates for Various Health Conditions:

One of the most remarkable aspects of Wall Pilates is its ability to be adapted to accommodate various health conditions. Whether you're managing chronic pain, recovering from an injury, or dealing with specific health concerns, Wall Pilates offers a safe and effective way to stay active and improve your overall well-being.

For women with chronic pain conditions such as arthritis or fibromyalgia, gentle, low-impact exercises can provide much-needed relief. Wall Pilates offers a supportive environment where movements can be modified to reduce strain on sensitive joints while still providing a challenging workout.

Similarly, women recovering from injuries, such as back pain or knee injuries, can benefit greatly from the therapeutic nature of Wall Pilates. By focusing on proper alignment, core stability, and controlled movements, individuals can rehabilitate injured areas while gradually rebuilding strength and mobility.

Women with specific health concerns, such as osteoporosis or pregnancy, can also find safe and effective ways to stay active through Wall Pilates. By working closely with qualified instructors who understand their unique needs, these individuals can modify exercises to ensure they remain within safe limits while still reaping the benefits of regular physical activity.

C. Testimonials from Women Who've Achieved Success:

To truly understand the impact of Wall Pilates, we turn to the stories of women who have experienced firsthand the transformative power of this practice. From overcoming physical limitations to achieving newfound confidence and strength, these testimonials showcase the profound effects that Wall Pilates can have on women of all ages and backgrounds.

Sarah, a busy mother in her forties, struggled with chronic back pain for years. After discovering Wall Pilates, she found relief from her pain and regained strength and flexibility she thought she had lost forever. "Wall Pilates has been a game-changer for me," she says. "I feel stronger and more capable than ever before, and my back pain is virtually nonexistent."

Emily, a retiree in her sixties, was skeptical about trying Wall Pilates at first. But after just a few sessions, she was hooked. "I never imagined I could feel this good at my age," she says. "Wall Pilates has helped me improve my balance, flexibility, and overall strength. I feel like a whole new person."

These stories are just a glimpse into the countless lives that have been touched and transformed by Wall Pilates. Whether you're a beginner or a seasoned practitioner, there's no denying the profound impact that this practice can have on women of all ages and fitness levels.

In the chapters that follow, we'll dive deeper into specific exercises and routines designed to target different areas of the body and address common fitness goals. But for now, remember this: whether you're looking to build strength, improve flexibility, or simply feel better in your own skin, Wall Pilates offers a path towards holistic health and well-being that is accessible to every woman, no matter where she may be on her journey.

In this chapter, we delve into a comprehensive array of illustrated step-by-step exercises tailored specifically for women seeking to enhance their fitness through Wall Pilates workouts. Each exercise is meticulously crafted to target key areas of the body, focusing on toning, strengthening, and sculpting for a well-rounded and effective workout routine.

A. Upper Body Exercises for Toning and Strength:

1. Wall Push-Ups: Begin by standing facing the wall with your arms extended at shoulder height.

Place your palms flat against the wall, slightly wider than shoulder-width apart. Lower your chest towards the wall by bending your elbows, then push back up to the starting position. Repeat for a set number of reps to tone your chest, shoulders, and arms.

2. Wall Plank: Stand facing the wall and place your hands shoulder-width apart on the wall at chest height. Step your feet back until your body forms a straight line from head to heels. Hold this position, engaging your core and upper body muscles to strengthen and tone.

B. Lower Body Exercises for Sculpting Glutes and Legs:

1. Wall Sit: Stand with your back against the wall and lower your body into a seated position, as if sitting in an invisible chair. Keep your knees bent at a 90-degree angle and your thighs parallel to the ground. Hold this position, engaging your glutes and quadriceps to sculpt and strengthen your lower body.

2. Wall Lunges: Stand facing the wall with your hands resting on the wall for support. Take a step back with one foot and lower your body into a lunge position, keeping your front knee aligned with your ankle. Push through your front heel to return to the starting position, then switch legs and repeat to sculpt and tone your glutes and legs.

C. Core Workouts for Achieving a Flat Belly and Toned Abs:

1. Wall Crunches: Lie on your back with your legs extended and your feet flat against the wall. Place your hands behind your head for support, then lift your shoulder blades off the ground and engage your core as you crunch towards your knees. Lower back down with control and repeat for a set number of reps to target your abdominal muscles.

2. Wall Leg Raises: Lie on your back with your hips close to the wall and your legs extended vertically against the wall. Place your hands palm down on the

floor for support. Keeping your core engaged, lower your legs towards the ground until you feel tension in your abs, then raise them back up to the starting position. Repeat for a set number of reps to strengthen and tone your lower abs.

By incorporating these illustrated step-by-step exercises into your Wall Pilates workouts, you can effectively target and tone your upper body, lower body, and core for a balanced and sculpted physique. Remember to focus on proper form and technique, and gradually increase the intensity as you progress in your fitness journey.

TARGETED WORKOUTS FOR WOMEN'S HEALTH

In the journey towards holistic well-being, the focus on women's health is paramount. Recognizing the unique physiological needs and challenges faced by women, tailored exercise routines can play a pivotal role in enhancing vitality and addressing specific concerns. In this chapter, we delve into targeted workouts designed to bolster women's health across different life stages, from pelvic floor strengthening exercises to postnatal recovery workouts, and from pre and post-menopausal exercise routines to exercises aimed at alleviating common women's health issues.

A. Pelvic Floor Strengthening Exercises:

The pelvic floor serves as a crucial support structure for the organs within the pelvis, playing a vital role in urinary and bowel control, sexual function, and overall stability. However, factors such as pregnancy, childbirth, aging, and sedentary lifestyles can weaken the pelvic floor muscles, leading to issues like incontinence and pelvic organ prolapse. Therefore, incorporating pelvic floor strengthening exercises into your routine is essential for maintaining pelvic health and function.

Begin with Kegel exercises, which involve contracting and relaxing the muscles of the pelvic floor.

These exercises can be performed discreetly anywhere, making them convenient for daily practice. Additionally, movements like bridges, pelvic tilts, and squats engage the pelvic floor muscles while also targeting surrounding muscle groups for comprehensive strength building.

B. Postnatal Recovery Workouts:

Pregnancy and childbirth exert significant physical demands on a woman's body, necessitating specialized exercises to aid in postnatal recovery. Postpartum women may experience weakened abdominal muscles, pelvic floor dysfunction, and altered posture, among other issues. Hence, prioritizing gentle yet effective workouts is crucial for restoring strength, flexibility, and function post-delivery.

Focus on exercises that promote core stability and pelvic floor rehabilitation, such as diaphragmatic breathing, gentle abdominal contractions, and pelvic tilts. Gradually progress to low-impact activities like walking, swimming, and modified Pilates exercises to rebuild muscular endurance and cardiovascular fitness. Emphasize proper alignment and mindful movement to prevent strain and facilitate optimal recovery.

C. Pre and Post-Menopausal Exercise Routines:

The hormonal fluctuations associated with menopause can bring about various physiological changes, including bone density loss, muscle mass decline, and metabolic shifts. Engaging in regular physical activity can mitigate these effects, promoting bone health, preserving lean muscle mass, and enhancing metabolic function.

Incorporate weight-bearing exercises like walking, dancing, and resistance training to support bone density and strengthen skeletal structures. Additionally, prioritize flexibility and balance exercises to mitigate the risk of falls and maintain functional independence. Tailor your workouts to accommodate individual preferences and abilities, ensuring consistency and enjoyment in your fitness regimen.

D. Exercises to Alleviate Common Women's Health Issues:

Many women experience specific health concerns, such as menstrual discomfort, hormonal imbalances, and breast health issues, which can impact their well-being and quality of life. While exercise alone may not cure these conditions, certain movements can alleviate symptoms and enhance overall resilience.

Explore gentle yoga sequences, such as restorative poses and gentle twists, to alleviate menstrual cramps and promote hormonal balance. Incorporate chest-opening exercises and lymphatic drainage techniques to support breast health and circulation. Consult with healthcare professionals or certified trainers to tailor your workouts according to your individual needs and goals.

CUSTOMIZING YOUR WALL PILATES ROUTINE

In the world of fitness, one size certainly does not fit all. We all have different bodies, capabilities, and goals. That's why when it comes to wall Pilates workouts, customization is key. In this chapter, we'll delve into the art of tailoring your wall Pilates routine to suit your individual needs, preferences, and objectives.

A. Creating a Personalized Workout Plan:

The journey to fitness begins with a plan. Crafting a personalized workout plan ensures that your wall Pilates routine is not only effective but also enjoyable and sustainable. Start by assessing your current fitness level, considering factors such as strength, flexibility, and endurance. Take note of any injuries or physical limitations that may require modifications to your exercises.

Next, define your goals. Are you aiming for weight loss, muscle toning, improved flexibility, or enhanced overall wellness? Be specific about what you want to achieve, as this will guide the structure and intensity of your workouts.

Once you have a clear understanding of your starting

point and objectives, it's time to design your plan. Consider factors such as frequency, duration, and intensity of workouts. Determine which Pilates exercises and variations align with your goals and preferences.

Remember to listen to your body throughout this process. Pay attention to how different exercises feel and adjust your plan accordingly. Flexibility is key, so don't hesitate to tweak your routine as needed to accommodate changes in your body or lifestyle.

B. Adapting Exercises for Different Fitness Levels:

Pilates is a versatile form of exercise that can be modified to suit individuals of all fitness levels. Whether you're a beginner or a seasoned practitioner, there are ways to tailor wall Pilates exercises to challenge your body appropriately.

For beginners, focus on mastering the fundamentals of Pilates before progressing to more advanced moves. Start with basic exercises that build core strength, stability, and body awareness. As you become more comfortable with the movements, gradually increase the intensity by adding resistance or incorporating dynamic variations.

Intermediate and advanced practitioners can deepen their practice by refining their technique and exploring more complex exercises. Experiment with variations that target specific muscle groups or challenge your balance and coordination. Incorporate props such as resistance bands or stability balls to add an extra layer of difficulty.

Regardless of your fitness level, remember to prioritize proper form and alignment to prevent injury and maximize the effectiveness of each exercise. If you're unsure about how to adapt a particular movement, consult with a certified Pilates instructor for guidance and support.

C. Modifying Workouts for Specific Goals:

Your wall Pilates routine can be customized to support a wide range of fitness goals, from weight loss to muscle toning to improved flexibility. By tailoring your workouts to align with your specific objectives, you can accelerate your progress and achieve meaningful results.

If weight loss is your primary goal, focus on incorporating high-intensity interval training (HIIT) principles into your Pilates routine. Integrate dynamic movements and cardio bursts to elevate your heart rate and burn calories more efficiently. Combine strength-building exercises with cardio intervals for a well-rounded workout that promotes fat loss while sculpting lean muscle.

For those aiming to tone and sculpt their physique, emphasize resistance training and targeted exercises that engage multiple muscle groups simultaneously. Incorporate Pilates principles such as control, precision, and concentration to ensure that each movement is performed with intention and purpose. Experiment with different rep ranges and resistance levels to challenge your muscles and stimulate growth.

If flexibility is a priority, dedicate time to stretching and mobility exercises that lengthen and elongate your muscles. Focus on deep breathing and mindful movement to release tension and improve range of motion. Incorporate dynamic stretches and flowing sequences to enhance flexibility and joint mobility.

Ultimately, the key to success lies in finding a balance that works for you. Listen to your body, set realistic goals, and stay consistent with your practice. With dedication and determination, you can customize your wall Pilates routine to achieve the results you desire and enjoy a stronger, healthier, and more vibrant life.

CONCLUSION

Congratulations! You've reached the end of "Wall Pilates Workouts For Women," and I hope this journey has been as enriching and transformative for you as it has been for me. As we conclude our exploration of Wall Pilates, let's take a moment to recap key points, find renewed motivation, and extend an invitation to further enhance our practice within a supportive community.

A. Recap of Key Points:

Throughout this book, we've delved into the incredible benefits of Wall Pilates. From its ability to build strength and flexibility to its gentle yet effective approach in addressing various fitness levels and needs, Wall Pilates has proven to be a versatile and empowering workout method. We've learned about proper alignment, breathing techniques, and how to modify exercises to suit individual abilities. Remembering these fundamental aspects will serve as the cornerstone of your continued progress and success.

B. Encouragement and Motivation for Continued Practice:

Embarking on a fitness journey, whether it's through Wall Pilates or any other form of exercise, requires dedication and perseverance. There may be days when you feel challenged or unmotivated, but remember how far you've come and the positive changes you've already experienced. Celebrate your achievements, both big and small, and use them as fuel to keep pushing forward. Stay committed to your practice, knowing that each session brings you closer to your goals and a healthier, happier version of yourself.

C. Invitation to Join a Community or Online Support Group:

While individual practice is valuable, there's immense strength in community. I invite you to consider joining a local Pilates class or seeking out online support groups dedicated to Wall Pilates. Surrounding yourself with like-minded individuals who share your passion for fitness can provide invaluable encouragement, accountability, and inspiration. Whether it's exchanging tips, sharing progress, or simply finding camaraderie in the journey, being part of a supportive community can elevate your experience and deepen your commitment to your practice.

In closing, I want to express my gratitude for allowing me to be a part of your fitness journey through "Wall Pilates Workouts For Women." Remember, this book is merely the beginning—a stepping stone towards a healthier, stronger, and more empowered you. Keep exploring, keep growing, and above all, keep moving. Here's to your continued success and well-being.

Wishing you strength, flexibility, and joy in every movement,

THE END